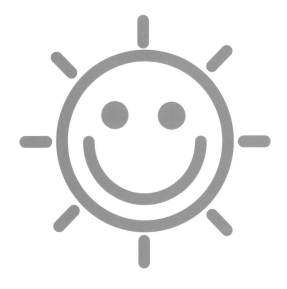

HEALTHY CHOICES

KEEPING CLEAN

Cath Senker

PowerKiDS
press.

New York

Text copyright © Cath Senker 2004
The right of Cath Senker to be identified as the author of this Work has
been asserted by her in accordance with the Copyright, Designs, and Patents Act 1988

Published in 2008 by The Rosen Publishing Group, Inc.
29 East 21st Street, New York, NY 10010

First Edition

Consultant: Jayne Wright
Design: Sarah Borny

The publishers would like to thank the following for allowing
us to reproduce their pictures in this book:
Corbis; 12, 14, 16 / Hodder Wayland Picture Library; 4, 5, 7, 8, 10
11, 15, 17, 19 / Zul Mukhida; 6, 9, 13, 18, 20, 21

Library of Congress Cataloging-in-Publication Data

Senker, Cath.
  Keeping clean / Cath Senker.— 1st ed.
     p. cm. — (Healthy choices)
  Includes bibliographical references and index.
  ISBN-13: 978-1-4042-4302-6 (library binding)
  1. Hygiene—Juvenile literature. 2. Health—Juvenile literature. I. Title.
  RA777.S39 2008
  613—dc22
                                    2007032793

Manufactured in China

Contents

Why do I have to wash?

Are you eager to be clean? It's great to feel clean and smell fresh. Washing yourself properly is very important. When you wash, you remove dirt and **sweat** from your body.

Dirt has **germs** in it. Scrub away the nasty germs at the sink or in a warm shower or bath.

Some parts of your body need washing more than other parts. Your hands and feet sweat a lot. You sweat under your arms and between your legs, too. Make sure you wash your hands, feet, and between your legs every day.

What things do you need to keep yourself clean and fresh? (Answer on page 23)

Why do I have to wash my hands?

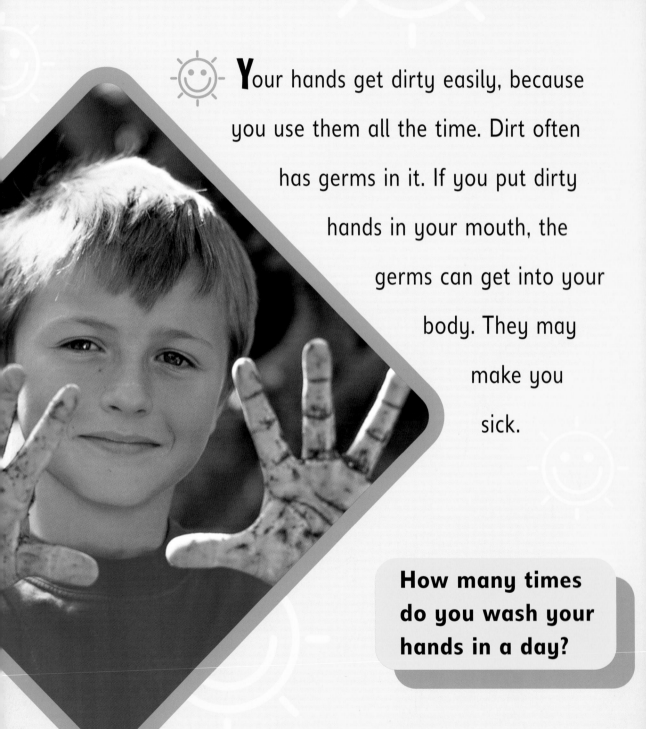

☀ **Y**our hands get dirty easily, because you use them all the time. Dirt often has germs in it. If you put dirty hands in your mouth, the germs can get into your body. They may make you sick.

How many times do you wash your hands in a day?

Germs are too tiny to see, so always...

WASH YOUR HANDS:

- after going to the toilet
- after playing outdoors
- after playing with pets
- before you eat

Make sure that you use soap and warm water to wash off the germs. Now it is safe for you to eat.

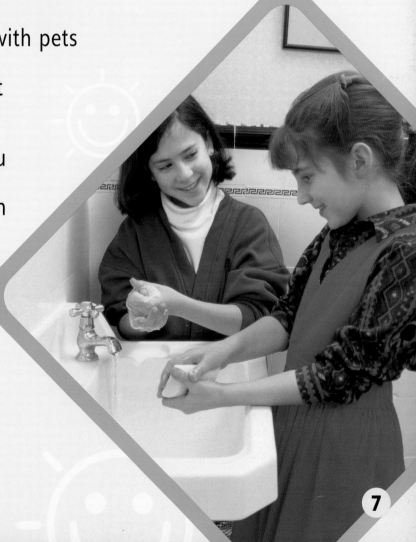

Why do I have to brush my teeth?

 You brush your teeth to clean off tiny bits of food. If you leave them, they can start to damage your teeth. That's why it's good to brush twice a day.

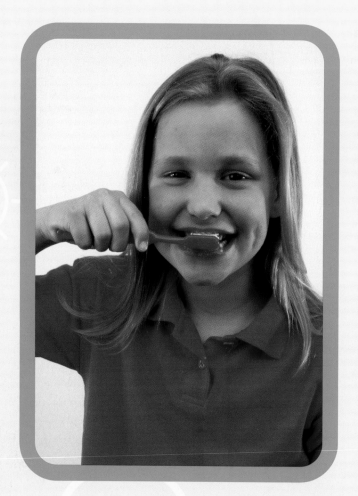

Don't rush when you brush. Clean the outside and inside of your top teeth. Clean the outside and inside of your bottom teeth. Then brush the tops of your teeth.

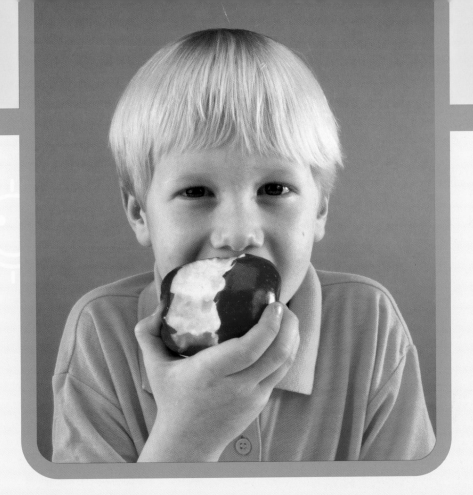

Remember to keep sweets just for treats. Keep your teeth happy with healthy foods, such as crunchy apples and juicy tomatoes.

List all the things you eat
and drink in one day.
Which things are good for your teeth?
Which things are not so good?

Why don't we wash our eyes?

 Your eyes are clever guys. They wash themselves!

When you blink, your **eyelids** spread tears over your eyes. This keeps them clean and *moist*. The tears wash dirt away. What happens if you try not to blink?

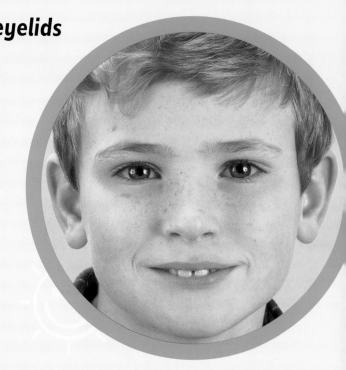

If you get something in your eye, don't rub it. You could scratch your eye and make it sore. Ask an adult to check it for you. Use plenty of fresh, cool water to clean out the dirt.

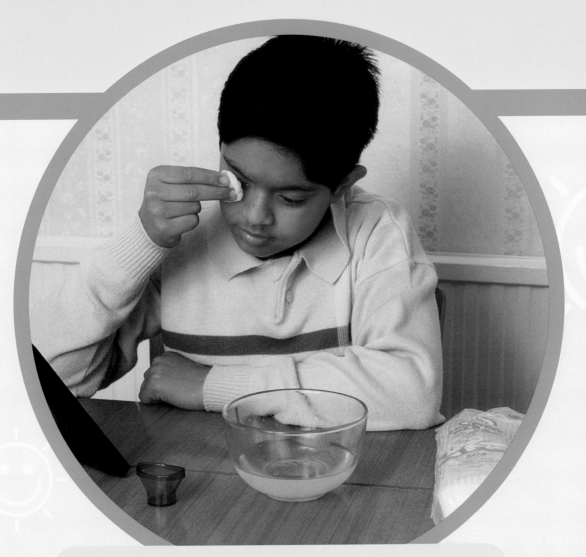

Use a damp cotton ball to carefully remove dirt from your eye.

Remember, you should never touch or poke somebody's eyes. Eyes are very special. They allow you to see the world around you.

How do I clean my ears?

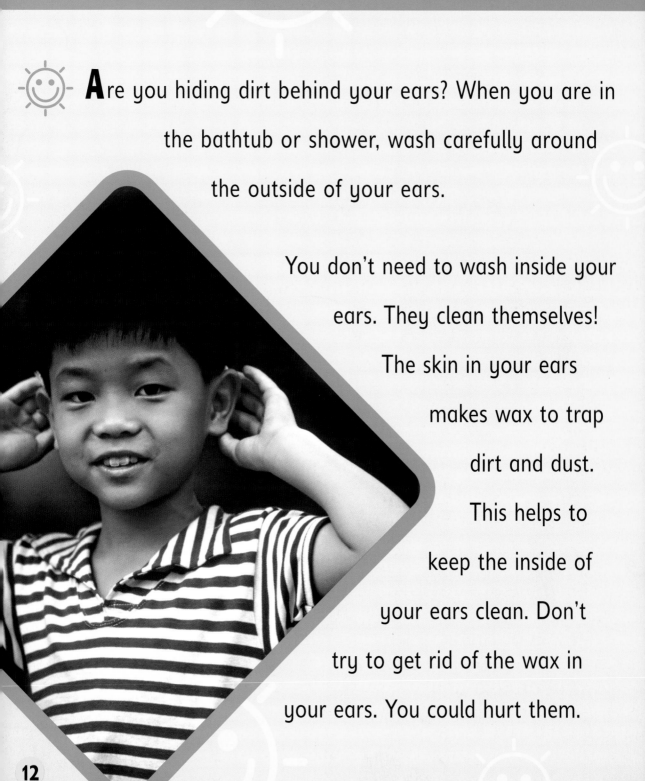

Are you hiding dirt behind your ears? When you are in the bathtub or shower, wash carefully around the outside of your ears.

You don't need to wash inside your ears. They clean themselves! The skin in your ears makes wax to trap dirt and dust. This helps to keep the inside of your ears clean. Don't try to get rid of the wax in your ears. You could hurt them.

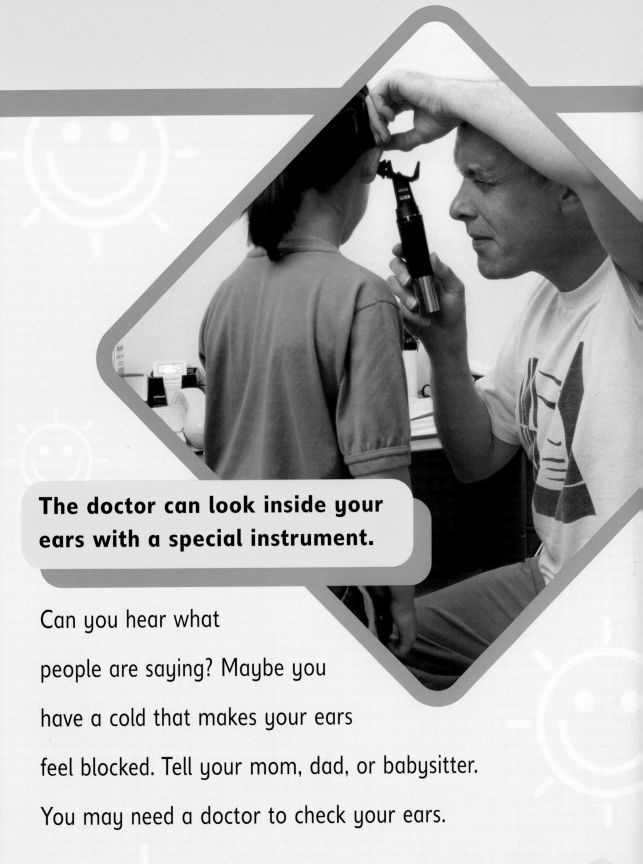

The doctor can look inside your ears with a special instrument.

Can you hear what

people are saying? Maybe you

have a cold that makes your ears

feel blocked. Tell your mom, dad, or babysitter.

You may need a doctor to check your ears.

Why can't I pick my nose?

 Inside your nose there is a gooey, slimy stuff called *mucus*. Mucus traps germs and dirt. It stops them from getting into your body.

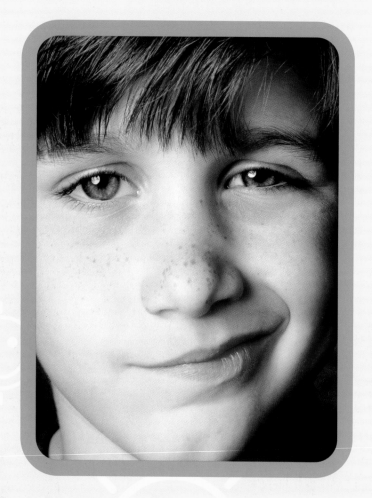

When you have a cold, your nose fills with mucus. The mucus stops the cold germs from getting into your body and making you more sick.

The mucus can make your nose run, or block it up. Don't pick your nose—use a tissue! Mucus is full of germs.

When you sneeze, try not to spray your germs all over your friends. Cup your hand over your nose and mouth. Use soft tissues to blow your nose—not your sleeve!

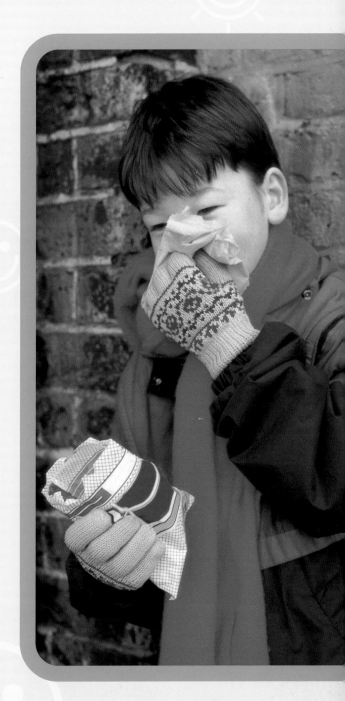

How do I take care of my hair?

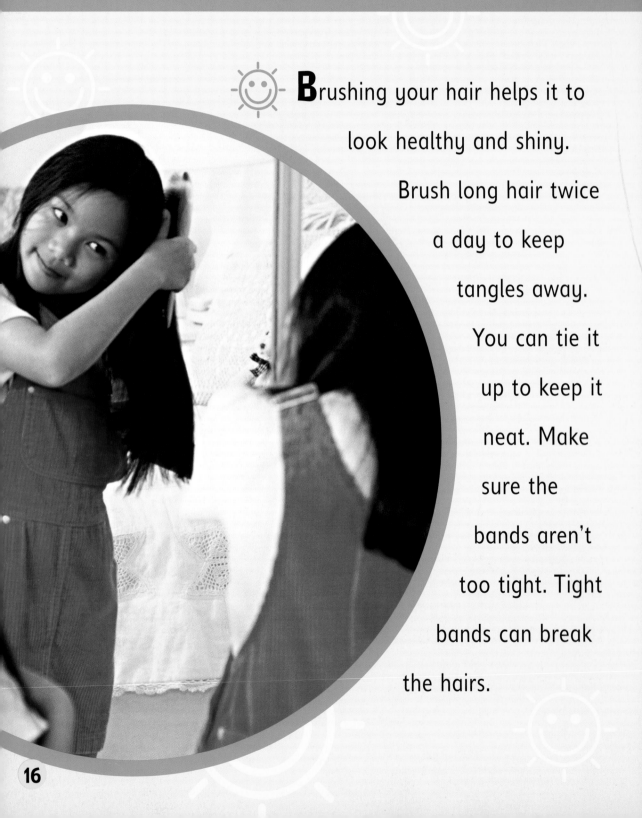

Brushing your hair helps it to look healthy and shiny. Brush long hair twice a day to keep tangles away. You can tie it up to keep it neat. Make sure the bands aren't too tight. Tight bands can break the hairs.

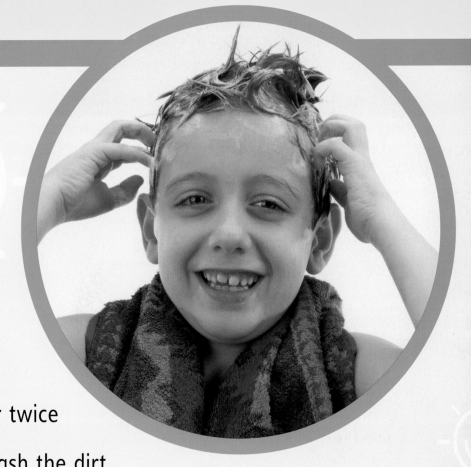

Shampoo

your hair at

least once or twice

a week to wash the dirt

away. Use a gentle shampoo and warm water. Some kids

like to use conditioner to make their hair easy to comb.

Always rinse your hair well with plenty of clean water.

Rub your hair gently with a towel. Carefully comb it,

so you don't damage the hairs.

What's wrong with biting my nails?

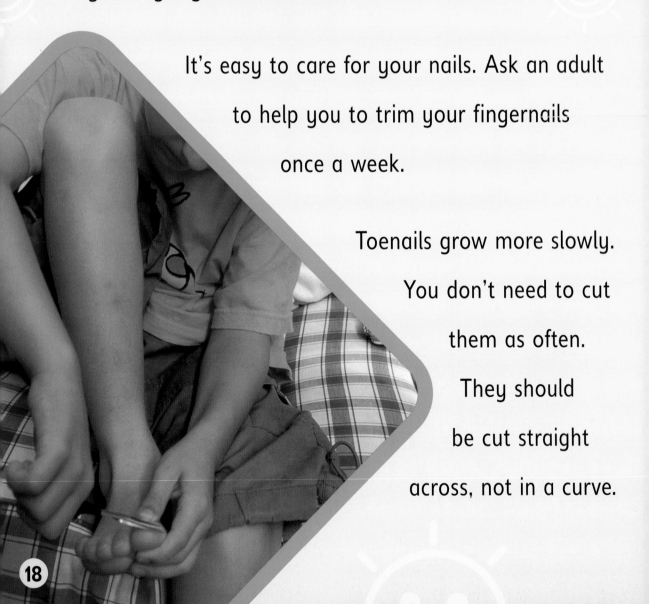

☼ **Y**uck! Try not to bite those nails. They're not always very clean. If you bite or pick a nail or **cuticle**, you might get an **infection**.

It's easy to care for your nails. Ask an adult to help you to trim your fingernails once a week.

Toenails grow more slowly. You don't need to cut them as often. They should be cut straight across, not in a curve.

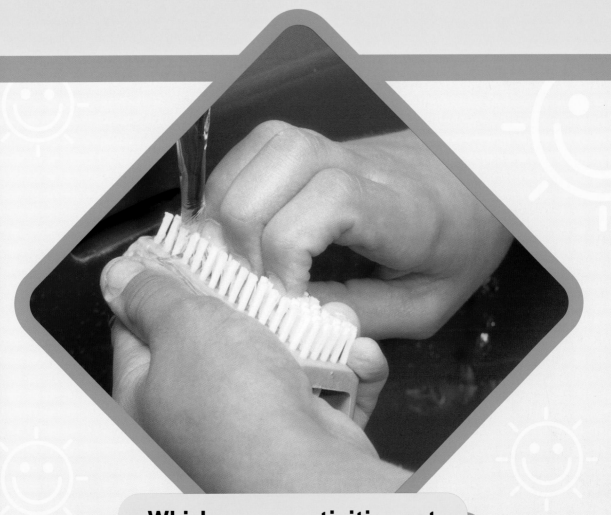

Which messy activities get dirt under your nails?

(Answer on page 23)

Dirt gets under your nails when you do messy activities. Remember to scrub them with a **nailbrush** when you wash your hands.

Can I wear my socks every day?

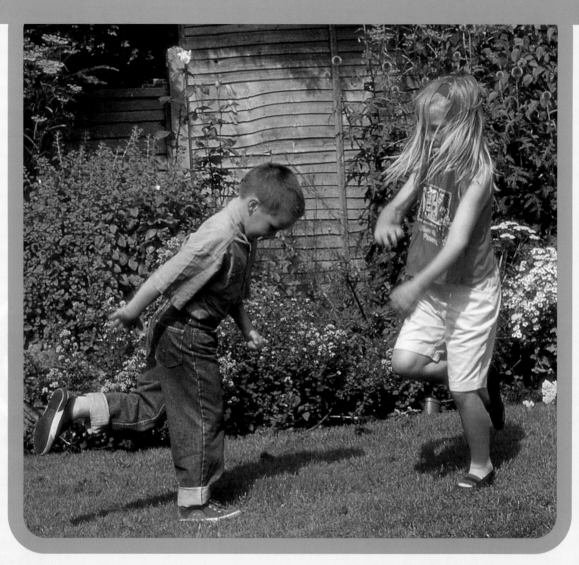

 Feet have to work hard, walking, running, jumping, and dancing. They get hot and they sweat. Your feet will get smelly if you keep wearing the same socks.

Do you have a favorite pair of gym shoes? You probably love wearing them. But it's better not to wear your shoes all day long. Feet love to be bare. Each day, give them some air.

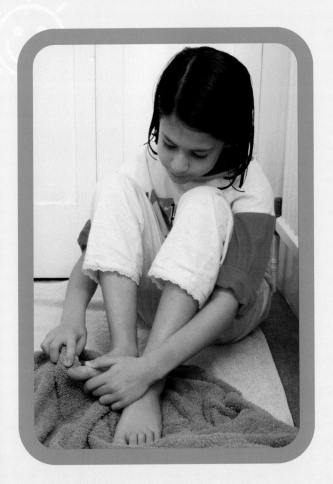

To keep your feet healthy, wash them at least once a day. Dry them very carefully on a fresh, clean towel. Change your socks every day. Make sure they are not too tight.

Glossary and index

Answers to the questions:

P.5   Some things you might need to keep clean and fresh are soap, bubble bath, shampoo, water, toothpaste, a toothbrush, a sponge, a washcloth, and a nailbrush.

P.19 Messy activities that get dirt under your nails might include playing soccer, gardening, playing with pets, painting, using modeling clay, and cooking.

Finding out more

Books to read:

Hygiene (What About Health?)
by Cath Senker (Hodder Wayland, 2004)

Say Aah! (New Experiences)
by Jen Green and Mike Gordon (Hodder Wayland, 2001)

Sophie's First Trip to the Dentist
by Michelle Lynn Rogers (AuthorHouse, 2006)

Splish! Splosh! Why Do We Wash?
by Janice Lobb, Peter Utton, and Ann Savage (Kingfisher, 2002)

Why Should I Wash my Hair and Other Questions About Healthy Skin and Hair
by Louise Spilsbury (Heinemann, 2003)

Why Wash? Learning About Personal Hygiene
by Claire Llewellyn and Mike Gordon (Hodder Wayland, 1998)

Web Sites
Due to the changing nature of Internet links, PowerKids Press has developed an online list of Web sites related to the subject of this book. This site is regularly updated. Please use this link to access this list:
www.powerkidslinks.com/health/clean